Copyright 2023

All right reserved.No part of this book should be reproduced without express permission of the author.

Reproduction of all or any part of this book is punishable unders relevant law.

1

Table of Contents

Interstitial cystitis (IC), often called painful bladder syndrome, is a tricky condition. It's tough to diagnose, and though treatments can make life with it better, there's no cure.

Because IC has such a wide range of symptoms and severity, most experts think it might be several diseases. If you have urinary pain that lasts for more than 6 weeks and is not caused by other conditions like infection or kidney stones, you may have IC.

No matter what it's called, interstitial cystitis symptoms bring a lot of challenges. The disease can affect your social life, exercise, sleep, and even your ability to work.

Despite this, you can still arm yourself with facts and treatments to keep symptoms in check.

BREAKFAST

1. Quesadilla with Refried Beans & Eggs

Prep Time: 10 Minutes

Cook Time: 15 Minutes

Servings: 3

Ingredients

- 3 large burrito size flour tortillas
- 1 cup black refried beans (or regular refried beans)
- 3 eggs
- 2 tablespoons butter
- Salt and pepper to taste
- 1 and ½ cup Mexican blend shredded cheese
- Sour cream, guacamole, and/or hot sauce, for serving

Instructions

1. On a large size non-stick skillet, melt 1 tablespoon of butter and scramble 3 eggs. Season with salt and

pepper. Set the eggs aside. We will use the same pan to cook the quesadilla.

2. Make a halfway cut on large flour tortillas from the center to the edge (cut a line from the center of the tortilla to the bottom edge). Gently fold the tortilla in 3 so it will leave folding marks to guide us where to put the fillings.

3. On the first area (the left side from the cut), spread ⅓ cup of refried beans evenly. Add the scrambled egg on top. Press gently on the eggs so they will stick to the refried bean.

4. On the rest of the area (⅔ of the tortilla), spread ½ cup of the cheese evenly.

5. Lift the side with the beans and eggs and fold it towards the second area. And fold once more to make the 3 layers.

6. Set it aside and repeat with the rest of the tortillas to make 3 quesadillas.

7. Heat the pan with ⅓ tablespoon of butter on medium heat. Add the assembled quesadilla to the pan. Cook until it is golden brown, about 2 to 4 minutes. Carefully flip the quesadilla and cook the other side for a couple more minutes.

8. Serve with sour cream, guacamole, and/or hot sauce.

Prep Time: 10 Minutes

Cook Time: 25 Minutes

Servings: 2

Ingredients

For smoked paprika garlic aioli:

- ¼ cup mayo
- 1 clove garlic, grated using a micro grater
- 2 teaspoons fresh lemon juice
- ¼ teaspoon smoked paprika
- Salt and pepper to taste

For tater tot breakfast hash (breakfast totchos)

- Half bag of frozen tater tots (about 14 to 16 ounces)
- 1 tablespoon oil, divided
- 2 eggs
- ⅓ cup caramelized onion
- 1 avocado, cut into bite-size pieces
- ⅓ cup red bell pepper (half of a pepper), sliced thinly
- salt and pepper to taste

Instructions

1. For smoked paprika garlic aioli (Make this first)

2. Mix all ingredients in a small bowl.

3. Keep in the fridge for at least 30 minutes to develop its flavor. It should keep in the fridge for up to 10 days.

4. For tater tot breakfast hash (breakfast totchos)

5. Cook the tater tots in the air fryer at 400F for 12 minutes. Shake and continue to cook for additional 3 more minutes.

6. While you are cooking tater tots, fry 2 eggs. Season with salt and pepper. Take the egg out of the pan once it is cooked to your liking.

7. On the same pan, add 1 teaspoon of oil and add the sliced red bell pepper. Season with salt and pepper. Cook for 2 to 3 minutes with frequent stirring. Set it aside.

8. Once the tater tot is done, assemble the breakfast hash. Add the tater tots to the dish that you are serving. Add the caramelized onion and cooked pepper on top. Place the avocado and cooked egg on top. Drizzle with aioli.

Prep Time: 15 Minutes

Cook Time: 30 Minutes

Servings: 7

Ingredients

For the pancakes:

- 1 cup all-purpose flour
- 2 tablespoons potato starch (or corn starch)
- 1 cup plus 2 tablespoons ice-cold water
- 1 teaspoon salt
- 1 teaspoon onion powder
- ½ teaspoon garlic powder
- 8 to 10 scallions/green onion, cut diagonally and thinly
- 1 carrot, cut into match sticks
- 1 small-size zucchini, cut into match sticks
- ½ medium-size onion, thinly sliced
- 3.5 ounces Enoki mushroom
- 7 to 8 teaspoons vegetable oil

For Dipping Sauce

- 1 teaspoon agave nectar (or sugar)
- 1 teaspoon Sambal oelek (or sriracha)
- 1 tablespoon soy sauce
- 1 to 2 teaspoon apple cider vinegar

Instructions

1. On a large bowl, mix together flour, potato starch, salt, onion powder, garlic powder, and ice-cold water until it resembles the pancake batter (it might be slightly thicker but not by much).
2. Add all the vegetables to the batter. Mix until all the vegetables are well coated with flour mixture. It may look like it is not enough batter but as time goes on, the water from all the vegetables will release, and the seasoning from the batter wilt the vegetable so it will be easier to work with.
3. In a small bowl, mix together all the ingredients for the dipping sauce and set aside.
4. On a small-size non-stick frying pan (I used 8-inch non-stick frying pan), add 1 teaspoon of vegetable oil on medium heat.

5. Add ½ cup of vegetable pancake mixture to the pan. By using a spoon, carefully spread the pancake mixture until it covers the bottom of the pan evenly.

6. Cook for 2 minutes. After 2 minutes, the edges should be brown. Flip them over and cook for an additional 2 minutes.

7. Take the pancakes out of the pan and add another teaspoon of oil. Remove the frying pan from the heat and add ½ cup of pancake mixture to the pan. Once you spread the pancake mixture evenly, return the pan to the heat and cook it for 2 minutes on each side.

8. Repeat until all the pancake batter is used up. You should end up with about 7 small-size pancakes.

9. Serve with dipping sauce.

Prep Time: 15 Minutes

Cook Time: 10 Minutes

Servings: 3-4

Ingredients

For sweet ricotta cheese:

- 1 cup ricotta cheese
- 1 to 2 tablespoons powdered sugar
- ½ lemon zest (optional but highly recommended)
- For French Toast:
- 1 to 2 tablespoons butter
- Half of the baguette, cut into a 1-inch thickness
- 2 eggs
- ⅓ cup milk of your choice
- ½ to 1 teaspoon cinnamon
- Pinch of salt
- 1 teaspoon vanilla extract
- 1 tablespoon sugar
- Fresh strawberry
- Fresh blueberry

- Maple syrup (for serving, optional)

Instructions

1. In a medium-size bowl, mix together ricotta cheese, powdered sugar, and lemon zest, if using. Transfer them into a piping bag or zip lock bag so you can use it as a piping bag. Set aside.
2. In a large shallow bowl, whisk together eggs, milk, cinnamon, salt, vanilla extract, and sugar until everything is well incorporated.
3. Coat the baguette in the egg mixture and let it soak for a couple of minutes.
4. In a large non-stick skillet, melt about ½ tablespoon of butter on low-medium heat. Add the baguette that has been soaked in the egg mixture. Cook for 2 to 3 minutes on each side. Repeat until all the toasts are cooked.
5. On a plate, place 2 to 3 pieces of french toasts. Add as much sweet ricotta cheese mixture and fresh fruits as you'd like. Drizzle with maple syrup (if using) and serve right away.

Prep Time: 5 Minutes

Cook Time: 10 Minutes

Servings: 4

Ingredients

- Medium size ½ onion, chopped (about ½ cup)
- Half of the red bell pepper, chopped (about ½ cup)
- Grapeseed oil, 2 tablespoons
- Roasted winter squash, 2 cups
- Kale (loosely packed), 4 cups
- ½ teaspoon Garlic powder
- ½ teaspoon smoked paprika
- Salt and pepper
- Fried eggs (optional)

Instructions

1. On a large skillet, heat 1 tablespoon of grapeseed oil on medium-high heat and sautéed onion and red bell pepper. Season lightly with salt and pepper, about 2-3 minutes.

2. Take the sautéed onion and pepper out of the skillet. Set aside.

3. On the same skillet, add the remaining oil and add the roasted winter squash. Cook until they are heated through and slightly browned, about 4-5 minutes.

4. Once the squash is heated through, add the cooked onion and pepper to the skillet as well as kale. Stir frequently.

5. Season the hash with garlic powder, smoked paprika, salt, and pepper.

6. Continue to cook for additional 2 minutes.

7. Serve with fried eggs and/or toast.

Prep Time: 20 Minutes

Cook Time: 80 Minutes

Servings: 5

Ingredients

- Acorn squash, about 1.5-2 lb
- Butternut squash, about 2.5 lb
- 2 Delicata squash, about 1.5 lb each (total of 3 lb)
- Olive oil spray
- Salt

Instructions

1. Preheat the oven to 400 degrees F.
2. Wash the winter squash under cold water.
3. Halve the winter squash lengthwise using a rubber mallet and a sharp knife.
4. Scoop out the seeds and pulps.
5. Cut the squash into the 1-inch strip. I cut mine against the rind (see the pictures above). For the butternut squash, I cut the round part (which enclosed the seeds

and pulps) into strip-like acorn and delicata squash. For the part where it didn't have any seeds, I peel the skin with a potato peeler and cut into 1-inch cubes.

6. Line the baking sheet with parchment paper and lay the cut squash on top. Spray with olive oil spray to coat and sprinkle some salt. Flip them over and do the same on the opposite sides.

7. Bake for 20 minutes.

8. Take the baking sheet out of the oven and flip the squash over. Bake for additional 20 minutes.

9. Take them out of the oven and let them cool to room temperature.

10. Once the squash is cooled, using a pairing knife, peel off the skin of roasted winter squash. Keep in an airtight container and keep it refrigerated.

Prep Time: 20 Minutes

Cook Time: 80 Minutes

Servings: 5

Ingredients

- 2 green onion, chopped
- 2 tablespoons grape seed oil
- 1 cup chopped kimchi
- 1 teaspoon sugar
- ½ teaspoon garlic powder
- 2 cup cooked rice
- 2-3 ounces of vegan soy chorizo
- ¼ cup kimchi juice
- 1 tablespoon sesame seed (for garnish)
- Snack size seaweed paper package, crumbled (optional)

Instructions

1. In a large skillet, add oil and chopped green onion and cook on medium heat until the onions are fragrant.

2. Add the chopped kimchi, soy chorizo, sugar, and garlic powder. Cook for 1-2 minutes.

3. Add the rice and kimchi juice. Stir frequently to mix everything well.

4. Continue to fry the rice for 3-5 minutes.

5. Turn off the heat and garnish with sesame seeds and seaweed paper.

Prep Time: 10 Minutes

Cook Time: 20 Minutes

Servings: 4

Ingredients

- 1 pound of Yukon gold potato, diced into ½ inch cube
- 1 teaspoon salt (optional, see note below)
- 4 ounces of vegan soy chorizo (⅓Soy Chorizo)
- ¼ large onion, diced
- 1 tablespoon olive oil, divided
- 1 teaspoon onion powder
- ½ teaspoon garlic powder

Instructions

1. Wash the Yukon gold potato and diced into ½ inch cubes. Place them into a medium-size pot and cover it with water. Add 1 teaspoon of salt (optional) and bring it to boil.
2. Once it comes to a boil, continue to boil for 5 minutes. Drain the potato and set it aside.

3. In a large non-stick skillet, cook 4 ounces of soy chorizo on medium heat for 3-5 minutes. The chorizo should crumble easily. Stir frequently with a wooden spoon. Once it's cooked, take them out of the pan and set them aside.

4. On the same skillet, add about ½ tablespoon of olive oil and cook the diced onion on medium heat until onions are translucent.

5. Add the boiled potato to the pan and add the rest of the olive oil. Season the potato with onion powder and garlic powder. Stir so the potato is well coated with the seasoning and oil.

6. Arrange the potato so that they form a single layer in the pan. Without stirring or touching the potato, cook for 3 minutes. This will brown the potato nicely.

7. Flip the potato and arrange them in a single layer again. Cook without stirring for additional 2 minutes.

8. Add the cooked chorizo and stir in with the potato. Cook for 1-2 minutes

Prep Time: 10 Minutes

Cook Time: 10 Minutes

Servings: 3-4

Ingredients

- 1 block of tofu (I use firm or extra-firm tofu)
- 1 tablespoon Nutritional yeast
- 1 teaspoon onion powder
- ½ teaspoon garlic powder
- ½ teaspoon salt
- ¼ teaspoon turmeric
- Black pepper to taste

Instructions

1. On a medium to large size non-stick skillet, place the tofu without any oil.
2. Smoosh/crumble the tofu with your hand. Gentle pressing of the tofu does the job.

3. Turn on the heat and cook for about 3-4 minutes until the water from the tofu evaporates. Stir frequently with a wooden spoon.

4. Season the tofu with nutritional yeast, onion powder, garlic powder, and turmeric.

5. Continue to cook for 3-5 minutes with frequent stirring.

6. Add the salt and pepper and cook for an additional minute or two.

Prep Time: 10 Minutes

Cook Time: 20 Minutes

Servings: 2

Ingredients

- 1 and ⅓ cup old fashion rolled oats
- ⅓ cup raw almonds, chopped
- 1 tablespoon ground flax seed
- 2 tablespoons coconut sugar
- 2 tablespoons coconut oil
- 3 tablespoons maple syrup
- 1 teaspoon vanilla extract
- pinch of salt

Instructions

1. Preheat oven to 325F.
2. Mix all dry ingredients in a big bowl.
3. Mix all wet ingredients in a small bowl.
4. Mix dry and wet ingredients together.
5. Line the baking sheet with parchment paper.

6. Lay the mixture in one layer and bake for 10 minutes.

7. Stir the mixture and bake for additional 10 minutes.

8. Let it cool completely and store them in an airtight container.

11. Vegan Hibachi Ramen Noodle with Vegetables

Prep Time: 10 Minutes

Cook Time: 10 Minutes

Servings: 4

Ingredients

- 1 small zucchini, seeds removed and cut into strips
- 1 small yellow squash, seeds removed and cut into strips
- ¼ teaspoon salt
- 2 instant ramen noodles (vegan) (use the noodles only and discard the sauce package)
- 1 tablespoon oil
- 8 ounces mushroom, sliced
- 2 tablespoon vegan butter, divided
- ¼ large onion, thinly sliced
- 2 tablespoons soy sauce
- 1 tablespoon vegetarian mushroom stir fry sauce
- Black pepper to taste

- Thinly sliced green onion and sesame seeds (for garnish)

Instructions

1. Remove the seeds of zucchini and yellow squash. Cut into thin strips lengthwise and cut into 2-inch pieces.
2. In a medium-size bowl, place a clean paper towel. Transfer the zucchini and yellow squash and sprinkle ¼ teaspoon of salt over them. Toss with your hands so the salt will even coat the zucchini and yellow squash. Set aside.
3. In a medium pot, boil water for instant ramen. Use the noodles only and discard the sauce package. Cook the ramen noodle 1 minute less than what it says in the instruction.
4. Drain and rinse the ramen noodle under cold water. Set aside.
5. On a large skillet, add 1 tablespoon of oil and cook the mushroom for a couple of minutes. Add a pinch of salt to help release the water from the mushroom.
6. Once the mushroom is wilted, add 1 tablespoon of butter and minced garlic. Cook with frequent stirring until it is fragrant, about 30-45 seconds.

7. Dap the water from the zucchini and yellow squash with a paper towel and add them to the pan with sliced onion.

8. Continue to cook for a minute or two.

9. Add the ramen noodle, soy sauce, and vegetarian mushroom stir fry sauce to the vegetable mix.

10. By using tongs, mix until everything is well coated with the sauce. Continue to cook for additional 2-3 minutes.

11. Remove the pan from the heat and add 1 tablespoon of butter. The heat from the noodle and vegetable should melt the butter.

12. Garnish with some black pepper, green onion, and sesame seeds. Serve right away.

Prep Time: 10 Minutes

Cook Time: 25 Minutes

Servings: 2-4

Ingredients

- 1 large size zucchini
- 1 medium to large size yellow squash
- ½ large red onion
- 1 cup and ½ cup cherry tomato
- ¼ cup + 2 tablespoons extra virgin olive oil
- ½ teaspoon salt + more to taste
- ¼ teaspoon ground black pepper
- 1 teaspoon dried basil
- ½ teaspoon dried thyme
- 6 ounces pasta (I used spaghetti), cooked according to package

Instructions

1. Preheat the oven to 400F.

2. Cut the zucchini and yellow squash in half, lengthwise. Then cut them into a half-moon shape, about ½ inch thickness. Cut the red onion in ½ inch thickness as well.

3. Transfer all the cut vegetables on a baking sheet pan and arrange them in one layer.

4. Drizzle about ¼ cup of extra virgin olive oil and sprinkle with ½ teaspoon of salt, black pepper, dried basil, and dried thyme on top of the vegetables.

5. On a smaller baking sheet, add the cherry tomato. Drizzle with 2 tablespoons of olive oil and season with salt and pepper.

6. Bake the vegetables for 20 minutes.

7. While the vegetables are baking, cook the pasta according to its package. Reserve about ½ cup of pasta water.

8. After 20 minutes, take the vegetable out of the oven. If you are making the pasta according to this recipe (for about 2-3 people), transfer half of the vegetables (not the cherry tomato) to a container. See the note for leftover vegetables.

9. Add the cooked pasta and roasted tomato to the baking sheet. Make sure to scrape all the oil and

tomato juice from the roasted tomato. Mix the pasta
with vegetables with tongs and enjoy.

Prep Time: 25 Minutes

Cook Time: 30 Minutes

Servings: 2

Ingredients

Sushi Rice:

- 3 cups cooked sushi rice (short grain rice)
- 1 tablespoon apple cider vinegar
- 1 tablespoon rice wine vinegar
- 1 tablespoon sugar
- ½ teaspoon salt

Spicy Mayo Sauce:

- 3 tablespoons vegan mayo
- 1 tablespoon sweet chili sauce
- 1 tablespoon sriracha

Sushi Bowl:

- 4 to 6 vegan fishless filets, cooked according to package
- ⅓ English cucumber, diced into small cubes

- 2 small avocados or 1 large avocado, diced
- 1 small green onion, thinly sliced (for garnish)

Instructions

1. Bake the vegan fishless filets according to their package.
2. While the fishless filets are baking, mix together apple cider vinegar, rice wine vinegar, sugar, and salt in a small bowl. Stir until sugar and salt are dissolved. Add the mixture to the cooked sushi rice. Set aside.
3. In another small bowl, mix together vegan mayo, sweet chili sauce, and sriracha. Set aside.
4. Assemble the sushi bowl. Place the seasoned sushi rice in a bowl, about 1 and ½ cups. Add the diced cucumber, vegan fishless filets, and avocado. Drizzle with vegan spicy mayo sauce. Garnish with green onion.

Prep Time: 30 Minutes

Cook Time: 15 Minutes

Servings: 8

Ingredients

- 6 cups cooked short-grain rice/sushi rice
- 2 tablespoons sesame seed oil
- 1 teaspoon salt
- 3 eggs
- 1 tablespoon Mirin (optional)
- 1 tablespoon vegetable oil, divided
- 2 carrots, cut into thin match sticks
- 3 king oyster mushroom, cut into thin match sticks (you can use any mushroom)
- 1 tablespoon dark soy sauce (you can use regular soy sauce)
- 1 teaspoon sugar
- ¼ teaspoon garlic powder
- Pinch of black pepper
- ½ English cucumber, thinly sliced
- Salt to taste

- 6 ounces of Korean pickled radish, cut into thin disks (optional) (see NOTE)
- 8 seaweed papers/Nori sheets

Instructions

For the rice

1. In a large bowl, mix together cooked rice, sesame seed oil, and 1 teaspoon salt until everything is well mixed.
2. Let the rice cool to room temperature.

For the fillings

1. In a medium-size bowl, whisk the eggs, Mirin, and ¼ teaspoon of salt together until everything is well mixed.
2. Cut the English cucumber into thin slices. Sprinkle some salt over This will draw water out of the cucumber and season the cucumber.
3. Heat ½ tablespoon of oil on a large non-stick pan. Add the egg mixture and swirl it around so the egg mixture will cover the bottom of the pan.
4. Turn the heat down to medium-low and continue to cook the egg until the edge is cooked. Carefully flip the egg over and cook the other side for a couple more

minutes. Take the egg out of the pan and cut it into strips. Set aside.

5. On the same pan, heat the rest of the oil and cook the carrot for a couple of minutes. Once the carrot is vibrant in color take them out and set them aside.

6. Thinly slice the Korean pickled radish and set aside.

7. By using a paper towel dab the cucumber so it can absorb the water.

For making onigirazu

1. Place the seaweed paper diagonally and the rough side up on the board.

2. Place about ⅓ cup of seasoned rice in the middle.

3. Place all the toppings on top of the rice carefully

4. Add another ⅓ cup of rice on top of the fillings.

5. Fold each side of the seaweed paper towards the center.

6. Fold the top and bottom corners of the seaweed paper towards the center while gently holding on to the layers.

7. Place your wrapped onigirazu folded side down. To secure and shape them further, wrap the onigirazu again with plastic wrap and let it sit for a couple of minutes.

8. Repeat until you use up the rest of the ingredients.
   You will make about 8 onigirazu.

9. Cut them in half and serve right away.

Prep Time: 10 Minutes

Cook Time: 15 Minutes

Servings: 6

Ingredients

- 6 sweet dinner roll, cut in half
- 4 tablespoons pesto of your choice
- 1 to 2 fresh mozzarella cheese balls, sliced
- 2 small tomatoes, sliced
- Salt and pepper to taste
- Red pepper flakes (optional)
- 2 to 3 tablespoons balsamic glaze

Instructions

1. Place the sliced mozzarella cheese on a clean kitchen towel or paper towel to absorb its access water.
2. Slice the dinner roll in half. Slice the tomato and set it aside.
3. Spread 1 teaspoon of pesto on the bottom of each roll.

4. Spread 1 teaspoon of pesto on the top part of each roll. Set them aside.

5. Place the sliced mozzarella cheese and tomato on the bottom of each roll.

6. Sprinkle with salt, pepper, and red pepper flakes.

7. Drizzle with balsamic glaze.

8. Top with the other half of the roll and serve right away.

Prep Time: 10 Minutes

Cook Time: 20 Minutes

Servings: 4

Ingredients

- ¼ cup raw cashew
- ½ cup unsweetened almond milk
- 1 tablespoon oil
- 1 tablespoon vegan butter (or use another tablespoon of oil)
- ½ large onion, diced
- 2 teaspoons ginger, minced or grated
- 3 cloves garlic, minced
- 1 teaspoon cumin
- 1 teaspoon garam masala
- ½ tablespoon curry powder
- ¼ teaspoon turmeric powder
- ½ teaspoon paprika
- ¼ teaspoon ground black pepper
- 3 tablespoons tomato paste
- 1 cup cauliflower floret

- 1 cup diced potato
- 2-3 small size carrots, cut into small pieces
- ½ teaspoon salt
- 1 cup water (or vegetable broth)
- 2 teaspoons Vegan Chicken Flavor Bouillon Powder (omit if using vegetable broth)
- ½ cup frozen peas
- Rice and/or naan for serving

Instructions

1. In a high-speed blender, blend together cashew and almond milk until smooth. Set aside.
2. In a large non-stick skillet, heat oil and butter together and add diced onion. Cook until onion becomes translucent.
3. Add the minced garlic and ginger. Cook until fragrant, about a minute.
4. Add tomato paste, cumin, garam masala, curry powder, turmeric, paprika, and black pepper. Stir until everything is well mixed and bubbles a little in the pan.

5. Add cauliflower carrot, potato, water, and vegan chicken flavor bouillon powder (or vegetable broth). Add the salt.

6. Bring the mixture to a boil and place a lid on top. Reduce the heat to medium and continue to cook for 5-7 minutes until the potato is cooked but not mushy.

7. Add the cashew almond milk mixture and frozen pea to the curry. Stir to mix and continue to cook for additional 2-3 minutes.

8. Serve hot with rice and/or naan.

Prep Time: 30 Minutes

Cook Time: 45 Minutes

Servings: 8

Ingredients

- 2 tablespoons extra virgin olive oil
- 6 tablespoons salted butter
- 12 ounces wild mushrooms, roughly torn
- Salt and pepper
- 2 cloves garlic, minced or grated
- 1 tsp dried oregano
- 1/4 cup all-purpose flour
- 2 cups whole milk
- 2 cups vegetable broth
- 2 cups shredded Emmi Raclette (provolone or fontina can be used)
- 1 cup grated parmesan cheese
- 2 cups whole milk ricotta cheese
- 2 (10 ounce) packages frozen spinach, thawed and drained
- 1/2 cup basil pesto, homemade or store bought

- 1 box no-boil lasagna noodles

Instructions

1. Preheat the oven to 350 degrees F. Grease a 9x13 inch pan.
2. Heat the olive oil In a large skillet over medium heat. When the oil shimmers, add the mushrooms and season with salt and pepper. Cook undisturbed for 5 minutes or until golden, stir and continue cooking until the mushrooms have caramelized, 3-5 minutes. Remove the mushrooms from the skillet to a plate.
3. Add the butter, garlic and oregano, salt, and pepper and cook 30 seconds or until fragrant. Whisk in the flour and cook for about 1 minute. Add the milk and broth. Bring to a boil and stir for 1 minute. Remove from heat and stir in the Raclette cheese and 1/2 cup of parmesan cheese. Stir until the cheese is fully melted and the sauce is smooth. Set the cheese sauce aside.
4. In a medium bowl combine the ricotta, spinach, and pesto.
5. Spread 1/4 of the cheese sauce in the bottom of the prepared baking dish. Top with 3-4 lasagna sheets.

Spread with 1/2 the ricotta cheese mixture, another 1/4 of the cheese sauce, and half of the mushrooms. Place another 3-4 lasagna noodles on top and then top with the remaining ricotta cheese mixture, another 1/4 of the cheese sauce, and the remaining mushrooms. Add the remaining lasagna noodles and pour the remaining cheese sauce over top. Top with a 1/2 cup of parmesan cheese. Bake uncovered for 45 minutes or until the top has bubbled up and browned a bit. Let stand 10 minutes before serving.

Prep Time: 15 Minutes

Cook Time: 25 Minutes

Servings: 4

Ingredients

- 8 slices thick sliced french or white bread
- 4 Tbsp butter, softened (salted or unsalted, whichever you prefer)
- 4 Tbsp mayonnaise
- 12-16 oz mozzarella cheese, shredded or thinly sliced
- 1 ripe avocado, sliced
- 1 cup baby spinach, leaves
- 4 asparagus spears, thinly shaved
- 1/2 cup micro green sprouts, (optional)
- 1/2 cup green goddess spread
- Green Goddess Spread
- 1/4 cup minced chives
- 2 Tbsp Minced fresh tarragon
- 1 garlic clove, minced
- 1/2 tsp anchovy paste, optional
- 3 Tbsp mayonnaise

- 1/2 cup packed baby spinach leaves, minced

Instructions

1. Make the green goddess spread: Mix all ingredients in a bowl until fully incorporated, set aside.

2. Mix the butter and mayo together in a small bowl. Spread 1 side of each piece of bread with 1 tablespoon (or more) of the butter/mayo mixture.

3. Heat a frying pan to medium-low heat. Place a slice of bread, butter side down in the pan. Top with 1/4 cup shredded mozzarella or thin layer of cheese slices (whichever you prefer). Top the cheese layer with 1/4 of the avocado slices, followed by 1/4 of the spinach, 1/4 of the asparagus, 1/4 of the sprouts and another 1/4 cup shredded cheese or more sliced mozzarella.

4. Spread 2 tablespoons of the green goddess spread onto the non-buttered side of one of the remaining slices of buttered bread. Place the slice of bread spread down on the sandwich in the pan.

5. Turn the heat to medium. Place a lid on the pan if desired to help trap the heat and melt the cheese. Flip when a golden crust is achieved on the bottom of the sandwich and the cheese is melted on the bottom.

Grill both sides of each sandwich and repeat 3 more times with remaining ingredients.

Prep Time: 30 Minutes

Cook Time: 15 Minutes

Servings: 10

Ingredients

- 10 mini brioche buns
- 1 lb ground beef
- 2 garlic cloves, minced
- 3 oz blue cheese, crumbled
- 1 tbsp worcestershire
- 1 tbsp dijon mustard
- 1 tsp salt
- 2 tsp freshly ground pepper
- 3 tbs olive oil
- sweet and spicy pickles (or store-bought)
- arugula
- toothpicks
- Sun-Dried Tomato Mayo
- 1 cup mayonnaise
- 1 tbsp lemon zest
- 1 tbsp lemon juice

- 1/2 cup oil packed sun-dried tomatoes, roughly chopped
- 2 tbsp finely chopped chives
- 3 garlic cloves
- 2-3 freshly ground pepper

Instructions

Sliders

1. To make the sun-dried tomato mayo add all of the ingredients in a small bowl and whisk until smooth. This can be made ahead and stored in the refrigerator for up to 2 weeks.
2. In a medium bowl, combing the ground beef, garlic, blue cheese, worcestershire, mustard, salt and pepper.
3. Using your hands form 10 patties 2-inches in diameter and ½ inch thick. Using your thumb make a small indentation in the middle of each patty.
4. Heat olive oil in a cast iron skillet over medium/high heat until just beginning to smoke. Arrange patties in the skillet so they are not crowded. (You may have to cook them in two batches.) Once the patties are brown on one side (about 3 minutes) flip them and cook on the other side for 2 more minutes. Once the patties

are cooked, transfer them to a paper towel lined platter and cook the second batch.

5. Toast the buns on a baking sheet cut side up on broil for just a few minutes until golden brown. Serve sliders on the buns with spicy pickles, arugula and sun-dried tomato mayo. Use a toothpick to hold together.

Prep Time: 20 Minutes

Cook Time: 40 Minutes

Servings: 8

Ingredients

Meatballs:

- 1 lbground beef
- 1 lb ground pork
- ¼ cup flat leaf parsley, minced
- ½ tsp ground allspice
- ½ tsp ground nutmeg
- ¾ cup yellow onion, grated (about 1 medium onion)
- 2 tsp salt
- ½ tsp pepper, freshly ground
- 4 cloves garlic, minced
- ¾ cup panko
- 2 eggs
- 2 tbsp olive oil
- Cream Gravy
- ½ cup butter

- ½ cup flour
- 4 cups beef broth
- 1 tsp salt
- ¼ tsp pepper
- 1 tbsp lemon juice
- ¼ tsp ground allspice
- ¼ tsp ground nutmeg
- 1 cup heavy cream

Instructions

1. In a large bowl, mix the beef, pork, parsley, allspice, nutmeg, grated onion, salt, pepper, garlic, panko and eggs until combined.
2. Using a tablespoon or cookie scoop, measure out the meat mixture into roughly 35 (1.5 inch) balls.
3. In a large pan, heat 2 tablespoon of olive oil over medium-high heat. Add ½ of the meatballs and cook until browned on all sides. This takes about 5 minutes. Set aside
4. When all of the meatballs are browned, pour off any excess grease in the pan, into a heatproof vessel. Lower the heat to medium and add the butter to the pan. When the butter begins to bubble, sprinkle in the

flour and cook for 1 minute. Add the beef broth to the pan a little at a time.

5. Whisk the gravy until the broth is all incorporated. Add salt, pepper, lemon juice, allspice and nutmeg. Whisk a few more times. Slowly add the cream.

6. Once the gravy begins to simmer, add the meatballs back into the pan.

7. Simmer until the gravy has thicken up a bit and the meatballs are cooked all the way through about 8-10 minutes.

8. Serve warm over mashed potatoes or egg noodles, alongside steamed veggies and lingonberry jam.

9. Cooking Notes:

10. Gluten Free Version: if you want to keep this recipe gluten free, you can sub the breadcrumbs for a gluten-free version. To keep the gluten out of the gravy, you will want to reserve 1 cup of beef stock and mix it with ⅓ cup corn starch. Add it to the gravy at the end to thicken it up.

11. I like to shape the meatballs and place them on a piece of parchment paper for easy clean up and less dishes. Then I use another piece of parchment to place the browned meatballs on, again, easy clean up, less dishes.

12. If you take your time adding the beef broth, your gravy will stay thick, taking less time overall.

13. Take care not to boil the cream. It might separate if you do. Keep it at a simmer until the meatballs are cooked all the way through.

14. The meatballs should reach an internal temperature of 165° F and no longer be pink on the inside.

21. Easy Chicken Ramen Soup

Prep Time: 15 Minutes

Cook Time: 15 Minutes

Servings: 2

Ingredients

- 1 tbsp Organic Sesame Oil
- 4 garlic cloves, minced
- 2 tbsp ginger, minced
- 6 cups chicken stock
- 3 tbsp soy sauce
- 1/2 bunch green onions, chopped
- 3.2 oz package shiitake mushrooms, sliced
- 1 cup cooked chicken, shredded or sliced
- 1/2 tsp salt
- 3 packs ramen noodles (flavor packet discarded)
- 2 6 minute eggs
- sesame seeds
- Scallion Chili Sesame Oil
- 1/4 cup Organic Sesame Oil

- 1 tbsp chili paste/ sauce
- 1/2 bunch green onions, chopped

Instructions

1. In a small bowl, combine the 3 ingredients for the Scallion, Chili, Sesame oil. Set aside.
2. Heat 1 tablespoon Organic Sesame Oil in a medium sized soup pot. Add the garlic and ginger and sauté until fragrant.
3. Add the chicken stock, soy sauce, green onions, mushrooms, chicken and salt and bring to a boil. Add the 3 packages of ramen (noodles only, discard the flavor packet). Boil for 2 minutes until noodles are soft. Remove from heat.
4. Sprinkle the sesame seeds over the soup and place the soft boiled (6 minute) egg in the bowl. Serve with the Scallion, chili, sesame oil.

Prep Time: 20 Minutes

Cook Time: 15 Minutes

Servings: 6

Ingredients

- 1 cup plain Greek yogurt
- 2 tsp cumin
- 2 tsp cardamom
- 2 tsp tumeric
- 2 tsp cinnamon
- 2 tsp salt
- 3 large boneless skinless chicken breast, sliced into 1inch strips
- 2 tbsp Extra Virgin Olive Oil
- 2 large red bell peppers, cut into 1/2-inch thin strips
- 1 purple onion, cut into 1/2-inch thin slices
- 1/2 cup peppadew peppers

Tahini Sauce

- 1 cup tahini
- 4 garlic cloves, minced

- 1/3 cup Extra Virgin Olive Oil

- 1/2 cup lemon juice

- 2/3 cup water

- 1/2 tsp salt

For Serving:

- 4-8 pita bread

- 1/2 english cucumber diced

- 1 Roma tomato, sliced

Instructions

1. Preheat the oven to 350°F.

2. In a large bowl combine the yogurt with cumin, cardamom, turmeric, cinnamon and salt.

3. Add the chicken to the marinade and toss until fully coated. Set aside.

4. Spread 1 tablespoons of olive oil onto a large rimmed baking sheet. Arrange chicken, onions, bell peppers and peppadews on the baking sheet and drizzle with remaining olive oil.

5. Place the baking sheet on the center rack and bake for 20 minutes until chicken is cooked through and onions and peppers are tender. If you would like the

meat and veggies to have a bit of char, broil for 3 minutes or until desired caramelization is achieved.

6. Prepare the tahini sauce by placing all ingredients in a medium sized bowl and whisking with a fork until smooth. It will look like it is seperating for a few minutes before it all comes together, this is normal!

7. Serve chicken and roasted veggies in pita bread topped with a generous amount of tahini sauce, cucumber and tomatoes. Enjoy!

Prep Time: 20 Minutes

Cook Time: 15 Minutes

Servings: 6

Ingredients

- 1 lb large, raw, shrimp, peeled, deveined, tail on
- 1 lb chicken sausage, fully cooked
- 1 lb asparagus, trimmed and cut into 3" pieces
- 2 medium shallots, sliced into wedges
- 1 Tbsp Extra virgin olive oil
- 1 tsp salt
- 2 tsp Old Bay Seasoning
- 1 lemon
- pepper, to taste
- Lemon Garlic Aioli
- 1 cup neutral oil (such as avocado or vegetable)
- 1 egg
- 1 garlic clove, smashed
- zest of one lemon
- 1 Tbsp fresh lemon juice, from 1 lemon
- 1 tsp salt

Instructions

1. To make the aioli, add the oil, egg, garlic, lemon juice and zest and salt to a mason jar. Place hand blender (also known as an immersion blender) at the bottom of the jar and turn it on. In a few seconds you will see the aioli start to form at the bottom. It will quickly begin to emulsify and become thick. Hold the blender at the bottom of the jar for the first few seconds until the oil has been incorporated, then move the blender up slowly until fully combined!

2. Heat oven to 400°F.

3. In a large bowl toss asparagus and shallots in olive oil with 1/2 teaspoon salt and spread on baking sheet along with sausage. Place on center rack and roast for 10 minutes.

4. Remove pan from oven and add shrimp. Season entire sheet pan with remaining salt, freshly ground pepper, old bay seasoning and squeeze the lemon over the top. Gently toss all ingredients on the pan and roast for an additional 6-7 minutes or until sausage is warmed through and shrimp is pink. Serve warm with the aioli. Enjoy!

Prep Time: 10 Minutes

Cook Time: 35 Minutes

Servings: 6

Ingredients

- 1 cup ketchup
- 1/2 cup brown sugar
- 1 1/2 tablespoons unfiltered apple cider vinegar
- 2 teaspoons Worcestershire sauce
- 2 teaspoons chili powder
- 2 teaspoons salt
- 1 teaspoon garlic powder
- 1 teaspoon onion powder
- 1 teaspoon paprika
- 1/4 teaspoon freshly cracked pepper
- 2 pounds boneless skinless chicken thighs, fat trimmed

Instructions

1. Preheat the oven to 425°F with a rack in the center position. Line a rimmed baking sheet with foil and set a metal wire cooling rack inside of it.

2. In a medium saucepan, set over low heat, combine the ketchup, sugar, vinegar, Worcestershire sauce, chili powder, 1 teaspoon of the salt, the garlic powder, onion powder, paprika and pepper. Whisk together to combine. Increase the heat to medium and bring the sauce to a simmer, then reduce the heat to medium-low and cook until the sugar has completely dissolved and the sauce is slightly thickened, about 5 minutes. Remove the sauce from heat. Reserve 3/4 cup of the sauce for serving.

3. Place the chicken in a large bowl and season it all over with the remaining 1 teaspoon salt. Add 1/2 cup of BBQ sauce and toss to coat evenly. Arrange the chicken on the prepared wire rack. Bake the chicken for 15 minutes, then remove the pan from the oven. Using a pastry brush, coat the chicken all over with half of the remaining bbq sauce, using tongs to flip over the pieces. Return the chicken to the oven for another 15 minutes. Remove and brush with BBQ sauce again, then turn on the broiler. Cook the

chicken until the edges begin to brown, 4 to 6 minutes. The chicken is done when the internal temperature reaches 165°F on an instant-read thermometer.

4. Serve chicken with the reserved BBQ sauce alongside.

Prep Time: 10 Minutes

Cook Time: 25 Minutes

Servings: 6

Ingredients

- 2 lbs gnocchi, refrigerated, shelf stable or frozen
- 1 large shallot or 1/2 red onion, cut into 1/2-inch thick pieces, or slices
- 1/2 lb broccoli florets from 3/4 lb head of broccoli, about 2 1/2-3 cups
- 1/2 cup extra virgin olive oil (always buy a good quality brand for pesto)
- 3/4 tsp sea salt
- 1/4 cup lightly packed basil leaves, plus more for garnish
- 1 garlic clove
- 1/2 cup grated parmesan cheese, about 1 oz
- Red pepper flakes, to taste

Instructions

1. Preheat the oven to 400°F. Place the gnocchi, shallots and broccoli onto a large rimmed sheet pan, taking care to keep them in their own separate sections, shallots on one end gnocchi in the middle and broccoli on the other end. Drizzle the whole sheet pan with 1/4 cup of the olive oil and sprinkle with 1/2 teaspoon of the salt, toss each section a little to completely coat in the oil, while still keeping them all sectioned out.Roast in the oven for 25 minutes until the shallot/onion and gnocchi are tender and the broccoli is browned on top.

2. In the base of a food processor, add the roasted broccoli along with the basil, garlic, 1/3 cup of the parmesan, remaining 1/4 cup olive oil and remaining 1/4 tsp salt, pulse until combined and nearly smooth with a little bit of texture still remaining. Scoop the pesto out and toss it with the shallots and gnocchi on the sheet pan.

3. Serve with remaining parmesan cheese, extra basil and red pepper flakes.

Prep Time: 20 Minutes

Cook Time: 15 Minutes

Servings: 8

Ingredients

- 2 lbs boneless skinless chicken thighs, cut into 1" pieces
- 1/2 tsp nutmeg
- 1 tbsp allspice
- 1 tbsp cinnamon
- 3 tbsp brown sugar
- 5 green onions, ends trimmed off and discarded
- 3 garlic cloves
- 1 tbsp paprika
- 1 tbsp salt
- 1 tsp black pepper
- 1 tbsp dried thyme
- 1/4 cup olive oil
- 1/4 cup fresh squeezed lime juice
- 1 cup cilantro, packed
- 1 red onion, cut into 2" pieces, divided

- 1 lb baby bell peppers, whole
- 1 pineapple, cut into 2" pieces
- metal or bamboo skewers, soaked in water for an hour

Instructions

1. In a blender combine the nutmeg, allspice, cinnamon, brown sugar, green onions, garlic, paprika, salt black pepper thyme, olive oil, lime juice, cilantro and 1/4 of the red onion about 1/4 cup. Blend on high until smooth.
2. Pour marinade over chicken and allow to marinate for 2-4 hours.
3. Preheat grill to medium heat.
4. On each skewer add chicken, pineapple, bell peppers and red onions, rotating ingredients evenly. Once prepared, place the chicken kebabs on the grill and cook until chicken is cooked through (registers 165°F on instant read thermometer), rotating often.
5. Serve with coconut rice!

Prep Time: 30 Minutes

Cook Time: 30 Minutes

Servings: 6

Ingredients

- 1 rotisserie chicken or 3-4 cups poached chicken
- 1 (15 oz) can fire roasted tomatoes, diced
- 1 (10 oz) can red enchilada sauce, mild
- 1 small onion, chopped
- 1 medium zucchini, sliced into 1/4-inch half circles
- 1 (4 oz) can green chilies
- 4 cloves garlic, minced
- 4 cups chicken broth
- 1 (14.5 oz) can creamed corn, undrained (can sub with 1 can sweet corn, drained)
- 1 tsp ground cumin
- 1 tsp chili powder
- 1 tsp sea salt
- 1/4 tsp freshly ground black pepper
- 3 bay leaves

Garnish

- 4 Tbsp chopped cilantro
- 1 lime cut into wedges

sour cream

- cheese, shredded (cheddar, mozzarella, Mexican blend)
- 1 large avocado, sliced
- Tortilla chips, crushed

Instructions

1. While rotisserie chicken is still warm, pick all meat of the bones, discard skin. Place the chicken meat in a large stock pot. Discard bones, or save if you like to make homemade stock.
2. Add to the pot the tomatoes, enchilada sauce, chicken broth, onion, zucchini, chilis, garlic, corn, cumin, chili powder, salt, pepper and bay leaves. Stir to combine and turn the heat to high.
3. As soon as soup begins to boil, turn the heat to medium-low heat and continue to cook, uncovered, until the onions are translucent and zucchini is tender, about 30 minutes.

4. Serve the soup topped with chopped cilantro, a squeeze of fresh lime juice, sour cream, cheese, avocado and corn chips.

Prep Time: 15 Minutes

Cook Time: 60 Minutes

Servings: 6

Ingredients

- 1/2 cup Dijon mustard
- 1/2 cup honey
- 1 1/2 tsp sea salt, divided
- 1 Tbsp apple cider vinegar (optional)
- 1 tsp paprika
- 1/2 tsp freshly ground pepper
- 3 tbsp Extra-virgin olive oil
- 2 large shallots, roughly chopped (about 1 cup)
- 1 lb fingerling potatoes (or yukon golds, cut into 1" pieces)
- 2 sprigs rosemary, stems removed, leaves chopped
- 1/2 lb green beans, washed and trimmed
- 2 lbs boneless skinless chicken breasts

Instructions

1. Preheat oven to 375°F.

2. Make the honey-mustard sauce: In a small bowl, combine the Dijon mustard, honey, 1/2 teaspoon salt, apple cider vinegar and paprika. Stir until smooth.

3. Season the chicken breasts with the remaining 1 teaspoon salt and the pepper.

4. Heat 1 tablespoon olive oil in a large oven proof skillet or braiser over medium high heat. When the oil is glistening, sear the chicken until golden brown, about 3 minutes each side. Remove the chicken from the skillet onto a plate.

5. Add the shallots and fingerling potatoes along with the remaining olive oil into the braiser and toss to combine. Sprinkle with rosemary and place the potatoes in the oven, uncovered, for 15 minutes.

6. Remove the skillet from the oven. Nestle the chicken (along with any juices from the plate) and the green beans into the par-cooked potatoes in the skillet. Continue cooking for another 15 minutes.

7. Remove the skillet from the oven and pour the sauce over the chicken, green beans and potatoes, toss to combine. Cook for 10-15 more minutes longer or until

the chicken has reached 165°F with an instant-read thermometer.

Prep Time: 4 Minutes

Cook Time: 20 Minutes

Servings: 4

Ingredients

- 4 cups cooked rice, preferably day old
- 3 large eggs, beaten
- 2 1/2 tsp toasted Sesame oil
- 1/3 cup Coconut aminos
- 1/4 tsp Salt, divided, plus more to taste 1/4 tsp
- 3-4 Tbsp Vegetable oil
- 2 medium carrots peeled and finely diced, about 1 cup
- 1/2 Medium onion, finely chopped, about 1 cup
- 3 Cloves garlic, minced
- 3/4 cup frozen peas
- 4 green onions, chopped
- 2-3 Tbsp soy sauce or Tamari

Instructions

1. If using freshly cooked rice (as opposed to day old) spread it out on a baking sheet or two large plates to cool.

2. In a small bowl beat the eggs together with ½ teaspoon sesame oil, 1/2 teaspoon coconut aminos and ¼ teaspoon salt.

3. Heat 1 tablespoon vegetable oil and 1 teaspoon sesame oil in a large saucepan or wok (if you have one) over medium heat. Add the carrots and cook for 3-4 minutes until slightly softening. Add the onions and cook for 4 minutes longer, until both onions and carrots are tender. Add the garlic to the pan and cook for 1 minute longer. Remove vegetables from the pan and set aside in a bowl.

4. Add 1 tablespoon of vegetable oil to the empty pan and quickly fry the eggs, moving them around until they're just set and there are no longer any wet parts. As soon as the eggs are cooked, take them out of the pan and add them to the bowl with the carrots and onions.

5. Add 1 tablespoon vegetable oil and 1 teaspoon sesame oil to the empty pan and fry the rice by spreading it in an even layer. Let the rice fry without disturbing it for

2-3 minutes at a time before tossing it and then frying it for another 2-3 minutes. Do this for a total of 3-4 times.

6. Add the carrot mixture to the pan along with the peas, eggs, green onions, remaining coconut aminos and soy sauce (or Tamari) to the pan and stir quickly over medium heat until it is all fully combined. Season to taste with salt.

7. We recommend cooking the rice at least 6 hours before making this dish or using day old previously cooked rice.

Prep Time: 14 Minutes

Cook Time: 10 Minutes

Servings: 5

Ingredients

- 4 cups brown rice, cooked
- 2 heaping cups broccoli florets
- 1 cup carrots, julienned
- 1/4 head purple cabbage, thinly sliced
- 6-8 large crimini mushrooms, sliced
- 2 tsp olive oil
- cilantro
- lime wedges
- Green Curry Sauce
- 1 cup raw cashews
- 2 tbsp green curry paste
- 14oz can coconut cream
- 1 tbsp lime juice
- 2 tsp fish sauce
- 1-2 tsp brown sugar
- 1/2 tsp salt

Instructions

1. To make the curry sauce, combine all ingredients in a Vitamix blender and blend on high until for 2 minutes.

2. In a small bowl, coat the mushrooms in the olive oil. Set a pot fitted with a steaming basket and 1 inch of water in it over low heat. Place the broccoli and mushrooms in the basket and steam until the broccoli is tender, about 5 minutes.

3. Assemble bowl by layering the veggies over the brown rice and drizzling with curry sauce. Garnish with Toasted coconut, cilantro and a squeeze of lime.

www.ingramcontent.com/pod-product-compliance
Lightning Source LLC
Chambersburg PA
CBHW061007260726
48661CB00005B/2095